Copyright© 2023 MSI Australia

All rights reserved.

ISBN: 978-0-6459403-5-0

Published by How2Books
Under licence from MSI Ltd, Australia
Company Registration No: 96963518255
NSW, Australia

See our website: www.how2books.com.au
Or contact by email: sales@how2books.com.au
Covers and Copyright owned by MSI, Australia

MSI acknowledges the author and images, text and photographs used in this book.

Published by How2Books

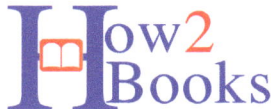

How2 Books

10% of the sale of each book helps to support Diabetes Type One and Cancer Research.

GRANDMA'S DIARY

YOUR DIARY/JOURNAL

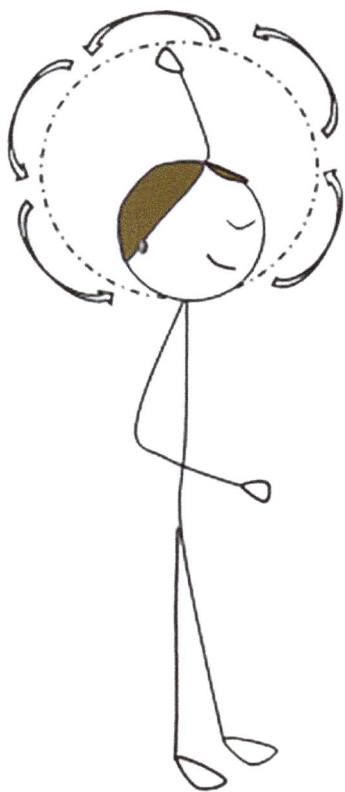

JANUARY

1)	Sunday
2)	Monday
3)	Tuesday
4)	Wednesday

JANUARY

5)	**Thursday**
6)	**Friday**
7)	**Saturday**
8)	**Sunday**

JANUARY

9)	Monday
10)	Tuesday
11)	Wednesday
12)	Thursday

JANUARY

13)	Friday

14)	Saturday

15)	Sunday

16)	Monday

JANUARY

17)	Tuesday

18)	Wednesday

19)	Thursday

20)	Friday

JANUARY

21)	Saturday
22)	Sunday
23)	Monday
24)	Tuesday

JANUARY

25)	Wednesday
26)	Thursday
27)	Friday
28)	Saturday

JANUARY

29)	Sunday
30)	Monday
31)	Tuesday

Your Notes

....

....

....

....

Your Notes

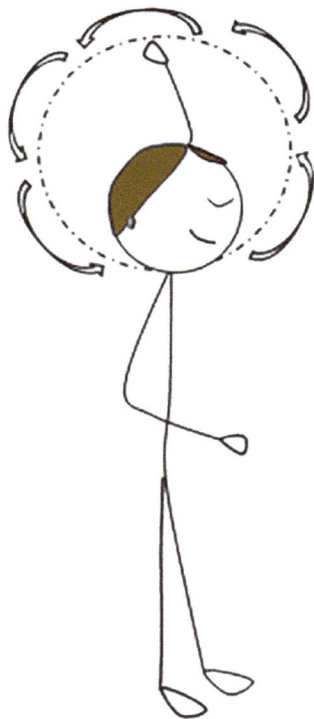

FEBRUARY

1)	Wednesday
2)	Thursday
3)	Friday
4)	Saturday

FEBRUARY

5)	Sunday
6)	Monday
7)	Tuesday
8)	Wednesday

FEBRUARY

9)	Thursday
10)	Friday
11)	Saturday
12)	Sunday

FEBRUARY

13)	Monday
14)	Tuesday
15)	Wednesday
16)	Thursday

FEBRUARY

17)	Friday
18)	Saturday
19)	Sunday
20)	Monday

FEBRUARY

21)	Tuesday

22)	Wednesday

23)	Thursday

24)	Friday

FEBRUARY

25)	Saturday
26)	Sunday
27)	Monday
28)	Tuesday

Your Notes

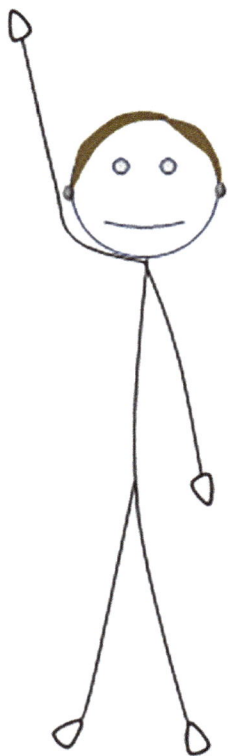

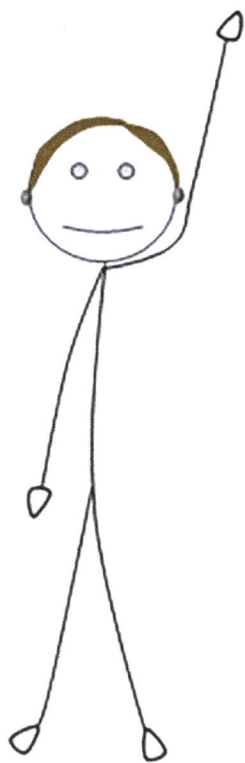

MARCH

1)	Wednesday
2)	Thursday
3)	Friday
4)	Saturday

MARCH

5)	Sunday
6)	Monday
7)	Tuesday
8)	Wednesday

MARCH

9)	Thursday
10)	Friday
11)	Saturday
12)	Sunday

MARCH

13)	Monday
14)	Tuesday
15)	Wednesday
16)	Thursday

MARCH

17)	Friday
18)	Saturday
19)	Sunday
20)	Monday

MARCH

21)	**Tuesday**
22)	**Wednesday**
23)	**Thursday**
24)	**Friday**

MARCH

25)	Saturday
26)	Sunday
27)	Monday
28)	Tuesday

MARCH

29)	Wednesday
30)	Thursday
31)	Friday

Your Notes

....

....

....

....

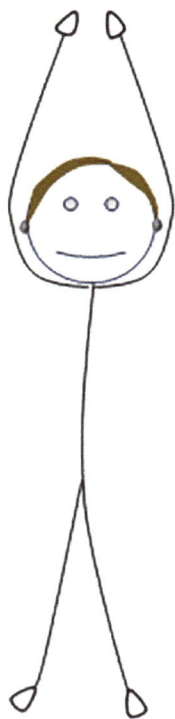

APRIL

1)	Saturday
2)	Sunday
3)	Monday
4)	Tuesday

APRIL

5)	Wednesday
6)	Thursday
7)	Friday
8)	Saturday

APRIL

9)	Sunday
10)	Monday
11)	Tuesday
12)	Wednesday

APRIL

13)	Thursday

14)	Friday

15)	Saturday

16)	Sunday

APRIL

17)	Monday
18)	Tuesday
19)	Wednesday
20)	Thursday

APRIL

21)	Friday
22)	Saturday
23)	Sunday
24)	Monday

APRIL

25)	Tuesday
26)	Wednesday
27)	Thursday
28)	Friday

APRIL

29)	Saturday
30)	Sunday

Your Notes

....
....
....
....
....
....
....
....
....

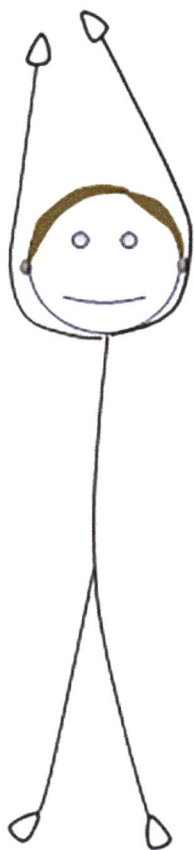

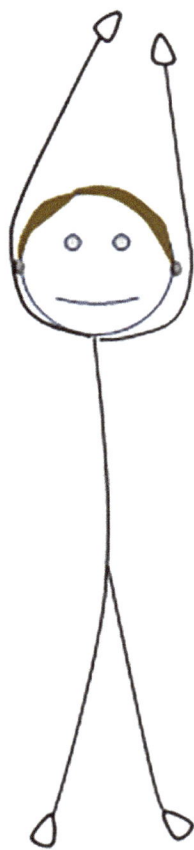

MAY

1)	Monday
2)	Tuesday
3)	Wednesday
4)	Thursday

MAY

5)	Friday
6)	Saturday
7)	Sunday
8)	Monday

MAY

9)	Tuesday
10)	Wednesday
11)	Thursday
12)	Friday

MAY

13)	Saturday

14)	Sunday

15)	Monday

16)	Tuesday

MAY

17)	Wednesday
18)	Thursday
19)	Friday
20)	Saturday

MAY

21)	Sunday
22)	Monday
23)	Tuesday
24)	Wednesday

MAY

25)	**Thursday**
26)	**Friday**
27)	**Saturday**
28)	**Sunday**

MAY

29)	Monday
30)	Tuesday
31)	Wednesday

Your Notes

....

....

....

....

....

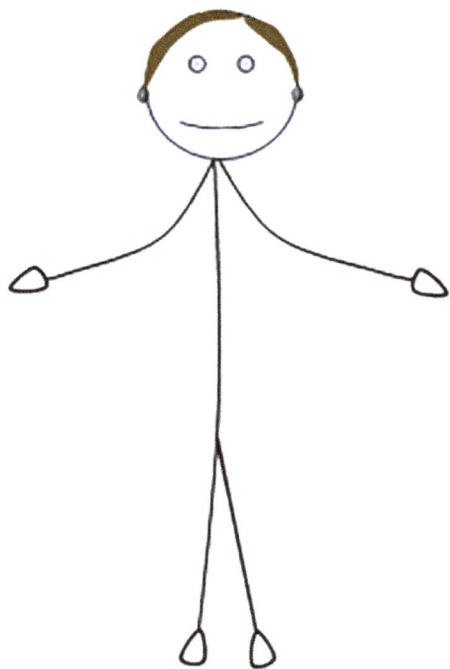

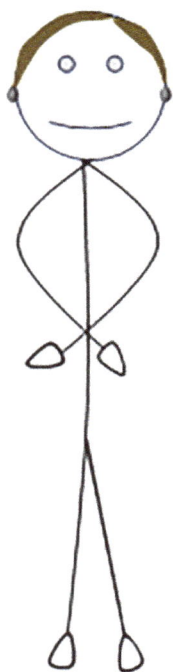

JUNE

1)	Thursday
2)	Friday
3)	Saturday
4)	Sunday

JUNE

5)	Monday
6)	Tuesday
7)	Wednesday
8)	Thursday

JUNE

9)	Friday
10)	Saturday
11)	Sunday
12)	Monday

JUNE

13)	Tuesday
14)	Wednesday
15)	Thursday
16)	Friday

JUNE

17)	Saturday

18)	Sunday

19)	Monday

20)	Tuesday

JUNE

21)	Wednesday

22)	Thursday

23)	Friday

24)	Saturday

JUNE

25)	Sunday
26)	Monday
27)	Tuesday
28)	Wednesday

JUNE

29)	Thursday
30)	Friday

Your Notes

....
....
....
....
....
....
....
....
....
....
....

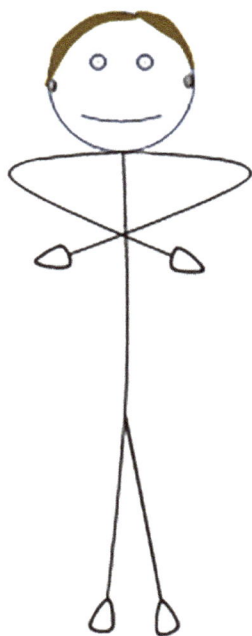

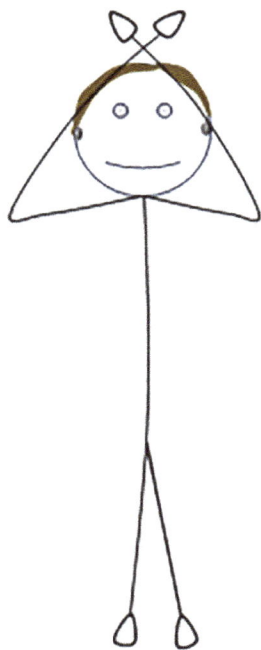

JULY

1)	**Saturday**
2)	**Sunday**
3)	**Monday**
4)	**Tuesday**

JULY

5)	Wednesday
6)	Thursday
7)	Friday
8)	Saturday

JULY

9)	Sunday
10)	Monday
11)	Tuesday
12)	Wednesday

JULY

17)	Monday
18)	Tuesday
19)	Wednesday
20)	Thursday

JULY

21)	Friday
22)	Saturday
23)	Sunday
24)	Monday

JULY

25)	Tuesday
26)	Wednesday
27)	Thursday
28)	Friday

JULY

29)	Saturday
30)	Sunday
31)	Monday

Your Notes

....
....
....
....
....

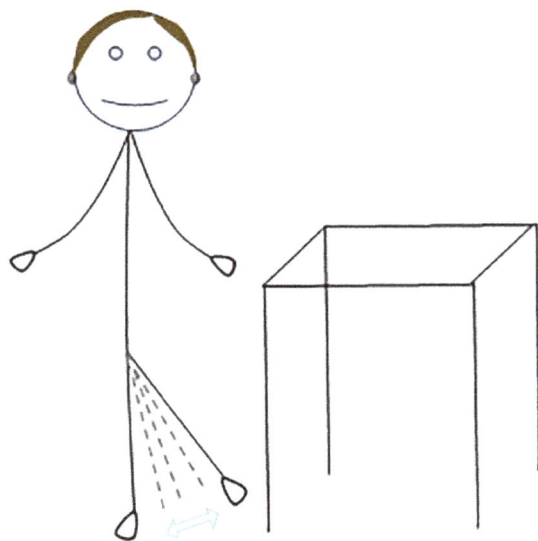

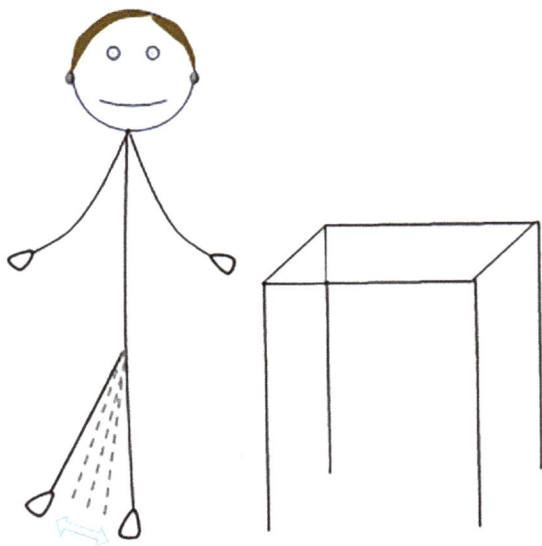

AUGUST

1)	Tuesday
2)	Wednesday
3)	Thursday
4)	Friday

AUGUST

5)	Saturday

6)	Sunday

7)	Monday

8)	Tuesday

AUGUST

9)	Wednesday

10)	Thursday

11)	Friday

12)	Saturday

AUGUST

13)	Sunday
14)	Monday
15)	Tuesday
16)	Wednesday

AUGUST

17)	Thursday

18)	Friday

19)	Saturday

20)	Sunday

AUGUST

21)	Monday

22)	Tuesday

23)	Wednesday

24)	Thursday

AUGUST

25)	Friday

26)	Saturday

27)	Sunday

28)	Monday

AUGUST

29)	Tuesday
30)	Wednesday
31)	Thursday

Your Notes

....

....

....

....

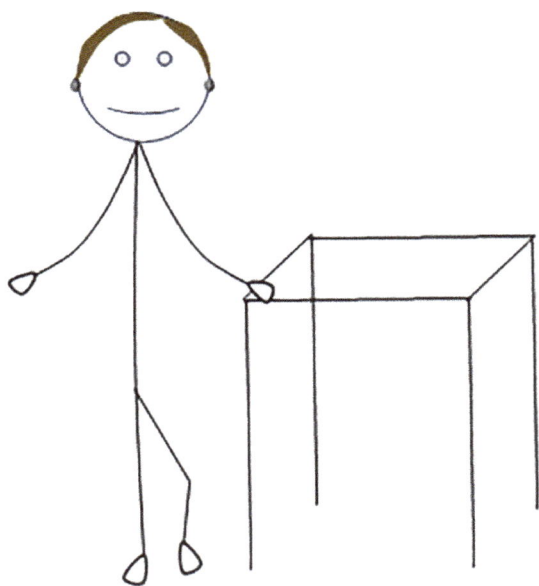

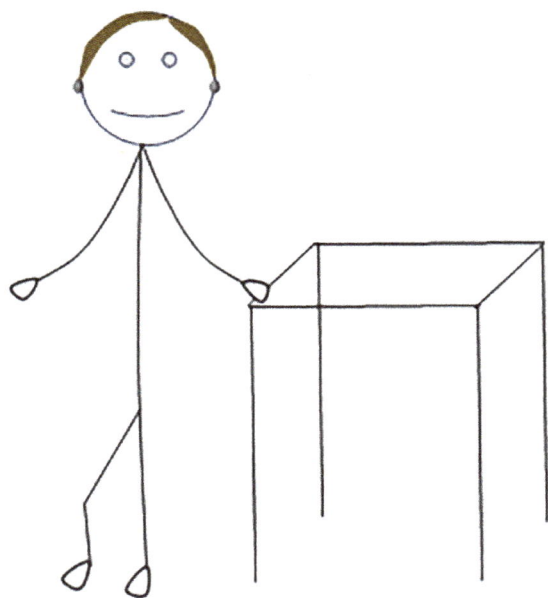

SEPTEMBER

1)	Friday
2)	Saturday
3)	Sunday
4)	Monday

SEPTEMBER

5)	Tuesday

6)	Wednesday

7)	Thursday

8)	Friday

SEPTEMBER

9)	Saturday

10)	Sunday

11)	Monday

12)	Tuesday

SEPTEMBER

13)	Wednesday
14)	Thursday
15)	Friday
16)	Saturday

SEPTEMBER

17)	Sunday
18)	Monday
19)	Tuesday
20)	Wednesday

SEPTEMBER

21)	Thursday
22)	Friday
23)	Saturday
24)	Sunday

SEPTEMBER

25)	Monday
26)	Tuesday
27)	Wednesday
28)	Thursday

SEPTEMBER

29)	Friday

30)	Saturday

Your Notes

....
....
....
....
....
....
....
....
....
....

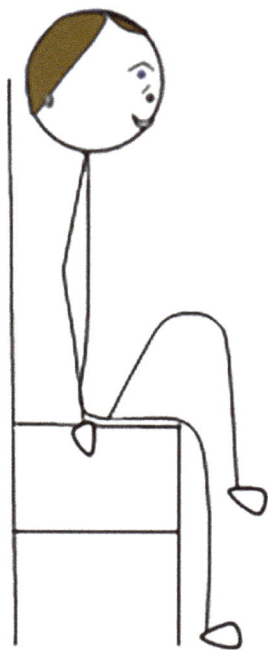

OCTOBER

1)	Sunday

2)	Monday

3)	Tuesday

4)	Wednesday

OCTOBER

5)	Thursday
6)	Friday
7)	Saturday
8)	Sunday

OCTOBER

9)	Monday

10)	Tuesday

11)	Wednesday

12)	Thursday

OCTOBER

13)	Friday
14)	Saturday
15)	Sunday
16)	Monday

OCTOBER

17)	Tuesday
18)	Wednesday
19)	Thursday
20)	Friday

OCTOBER

21)	Saturday

22)	Sunday

23)	Monday

24)	Tuesday

OCTOBER

25)	Wednesday

26)	Thursday

27)	Friday

28)	Saturday

OCTOBER

29)	Sunday
30)	Monday
31)	Tuesday

Your Notes

....

....

....

....

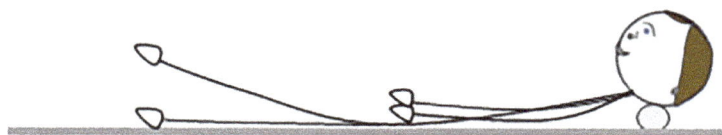

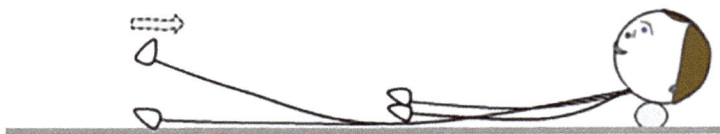

NOVEMBER

1)	Wednesday
2)	Thursday
3)	Friday
4)	Saturday

NOVEMBER

5)	Sunday
6)	Monday
7)	Tuesday
8)	Wednesday

NOVEMBER

9)	Thursday
10)	Friday
11)	Saturday
12)	Sunday

NOVEMBER

13)	Monday
14)	Tuesday
15)	Wednesday
16)	Thursday

NOVEMBER

17)	Friday
18)	Saturday
19)	Sunday
20)	Monday

NOVEMBER

21)	**Tuesday**
22)	**Wednesday**
23)	**Thursday**
24)	**Friday**

NOVEMBER

25)	Saturday

26)	Sunday

27)	Monday

28)	Tuesday

NOVEMBER

29)	Wednesday
30)	Thursday

Your Notes

....
....
....
....
....
....
....
....
....
....

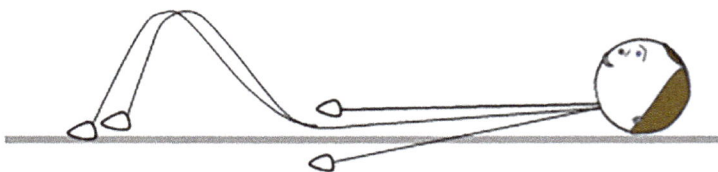

DECEMBER

1)	Friday
2)	Saturday
3)	Sunday
4)	Monday

DECEMBER

5)	Tuesday

6)	Wednesday

7)	Thursday

8)	Friday

DECEMBER

9)	Saturday
10)	Sunday
11)	Monday
12)	Tuesday

DECEMBER

13)	Wednesday
14)	Thursday
15)	Friday
16)	Saturday

DECEMBER

17)	Sunday
18)	Monday
19)	Tuesday
20)	Wednesday

DECEMBER

21)	Thursday

22)	Friday

23)	Saturday

24)	Sunday

DECEMBER

25)	Monday
26)	Tuesday
27)	Wednesday
28)	Thursday

DECEMBER

29)	Friday

30)	Saturday

31)	Sunday

Your Notes

....

....

....

....

....

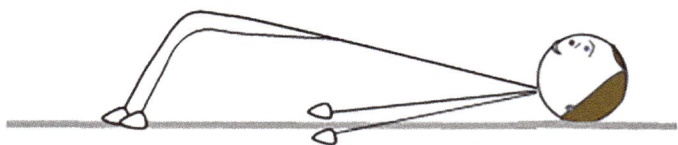